Massage & a Facial
Every 3,000 Miles

Also By Phebe Thorne

Camp Cooking in the Adirondacks

Massage & a Facial Every 3,000 Miles

A Roadmap to Looking and Feeling Good

Phebe Thorne

Illustrations by Nip Rogers

iUniverse, Inc.
New York   Bloomington

Massage and a Facial Every 3,000 Miles
A Roadmap to Looking and Feeling Good

iUniverse books may be ordered through booksellers or by contacting:

*iUniverse
1663 Liberty Drive
Bloomington, IN 47403
www.iuniverse.com
1-800-Authors (1-800-288-4677)*

*ISBN: 978-1-440-11147-1 (pbk)
ISBN: 978-1-440-11148-8 (ebk)*

Printed in the United States of America

iUniverse rev. date: 11/21/2008

*For my daughter, Helena, who encouraged
me to write this book and then helped
me get started. She is beautiful and,
of course, lives by these rules.*

Contents

Massage & a Facial

Every 3,000 Miles

Forward

Phebe is best described as a locomotive. She overflows with energy, power, and creativity from the moment she wakes up every morning (at 6AM, without an alarm clock) until extinguishing her light each night. She looks amazing – far better than you think a senior citizen might.

"10 Rules: Look Good, Feel Good" was a concept born around the dinner table. Friends and guests at her Adirondack camp, *The Uplands,* would marvel at her youthful appearance and consistently ask her: "What's your secret? How do you do it?"

For Phebe, the answer is simple, and so she easily sculpted her "secrets" into ten simple rules that amount to what she calls her Fountain of Youth.

It wasn't long ago that she found herself writing out these rules on a regular basis. And so, with her omnipresent determination and inherent desire to share her love of life with her friends, family, and everyone else, Phebe compiled the rules and their explanations into this little tome of reference.

~ Helena Marrin

Introduction

You've got to take care of what you have. Your body is the packaging for your spirit. If you abuse your body, it will die early and slowly, and your spirit will have no place to abide.

I have seen otherwise healthy people – people with no cancer or diabetes or other long-term health problems – who look awful. This makes them *feel* awful.

Who wants to look at a wreck every time they pass a mirror?

Taking care of yourself is not an absolute guarantee of perfect health or an insurance policy for a long life. Even beautiful, fit, well kept bodies can and do get cancer. Even thin people can get diabetes. Genes play a part as well as bad luck and exposure to various chemicals.

However, if you follow the ten rules I explain in this book, you will not only look good and feel good, your life will be more exuberant and happy. I can say with certainty that that is what has happened to me.

Most people I meet are not afraid to tell me that they are astonished to find out that I'm in my late sixties. Many people ask me how I do it. I had my daughter when I was forty, which has kept me active, but I attribute most of my energy and youthfulness to the following ten simple rules for overall health and wellness on the inside and the outside.

I call it my Fountain of Youth.

Phebe Thorne

April 2008

The 10 Rules for Looking Good and Feeling Good

1.   **Drink very little alcohol.**
2.   **Exercise the mind and the body.**
3.   **Allow yourself only a touch of sun.**
4.   **Get plenty of sleep.**
5.   **Eat good food.**
6.   **Meditate, practice yoga, pray.**
7.   **Love & Sex**
8.   **Have a massage and a facial every 3,000 miles.**
9.   **Laugh often.**
10.   **Do not smoke.**

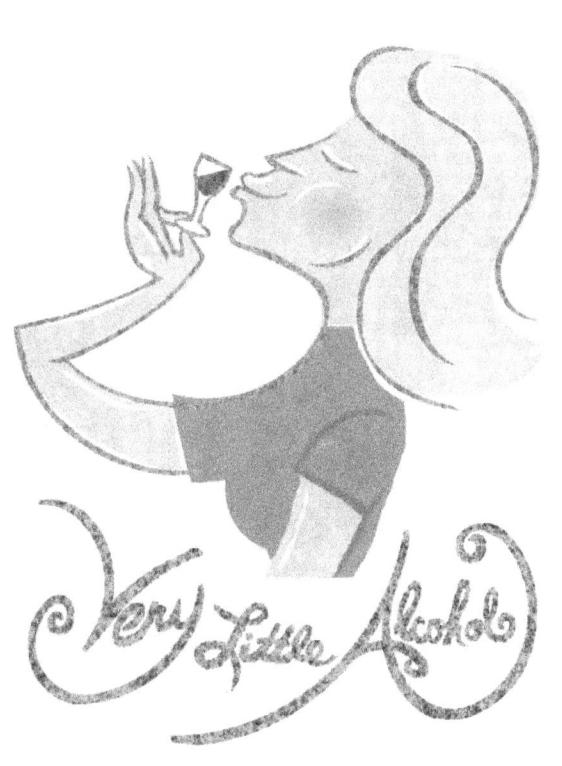

Rule #1

Drink Very Little Alcohol

Some alcohol has beneficial qualities. Red wine has flavonoid phenolics, which studies have found exhibit antioxidant and anti-coagulative qualities, thereby helping to prevent tumor growth and blood clots. Alcohol in general causes the capillaries to dilate so blood flow increases, particularly to the fingers and toes. It helps digestive juices flow, setting up a good appetite, and it aides in the processing of nutrients. Alcohol can also facilitate relaxation.

But too much alcohol is detrimental to your health and well being. The carbohydrates in alcoholic drinks will satiate you temporarily but won't feed you. Too much alcohol will kill brain and nerve cells and make you a bumbling idiot. Too much alcohol can obliterate liver cells, which can result in jaundice and cirrhosis.

Liver failure is no fun.

The liver is your filtering system and you die without it. Too much alcohol causes small blood vessels to break.

Notice the red noses and splotchy cheeks of people who drink too much? Those are all tiny blood vessels that have exploded – this is also what is happening in the brain and nerve cells!

Too much alcohol also causes dehydration. The headache that many experience as the most common hangover symptom is attributed mainly to a lack of necessary fluid intake. Fluids in the body are depleted by drinking too much alcohol, and a thirsty body is an unhappy body.

Fructose can help the body metabolize alcohol, so a rum punch is easier on your body than a shot of rum on its own. The higher the alcohol content, the harder it is for your body to cope. Hard alcohol is tough stuff; beer and wine are easier to metabolize. Moderate intake of wine (i.e. one four-ounce serving per day for women) might actually be beneficial. Just keep in mind that an excess of alcohol makes you look and feel awful the next day anyway.

Why bother?

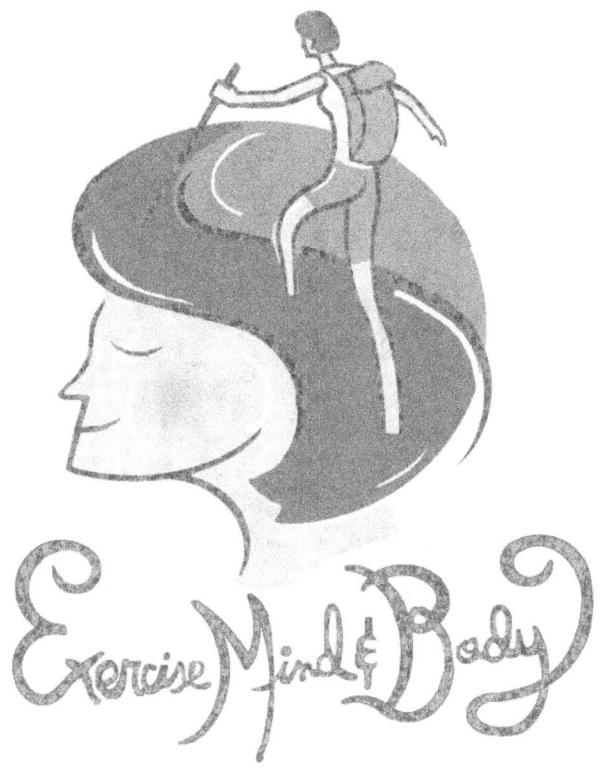

Rule #2

Exercise the Mind and the Body

Our bodies were created to excel at hunting and farming. As we sit in offices, cars, and on airplanes, we need to find ways to exercise, move, and get the blood flowing. The flesh deteriorates with inactivity. Muscle turns to flab or fat. Of course, flab and fat weigh less than muscle – a very pleasing thing at first, but don't be fooled. Muscle weighs more but takes up less room, and the more muscle you have the more calories you burn. If muscle tone is not there to support your circulation and your bone structure, your heart muscles weaken and all of a sudden a sedentary life becomes life threatening.

I have a close friend of the past fifty years who was so beautiful at age 19 and 20 that people thought she was a movie star. Even better, she had brain power superior to her looks. Sadly, her mother demeaned her intelligence and never praised an A on a math test or a term paper – she only wanted to know what dress her daughter would wear to the next party. For fifty years my friend has systematically destroyed her body in the hopes that people will judge her for her intelligent mind, not her beauty. What a shame, she could be loved for both.

It is important, however, not to go to the other extreme and become an exercise fanatic. Your body needs balance.

Allow your mind to flex its muscles. Do math problems – everyday finances are a good start. Read good books. Get involved in community activities and problem solve. Join a book club or investment club to keep you motivated. Exercise both your mental and physical muscles to obtain and maintain strength and flexibility.

New studies show that keeping your mind and body active help prevent Alzheimer's disease and dementia. The ancient Greeks knew there was something to it when they said: "Healthy mind, healthy body."

So exercise.

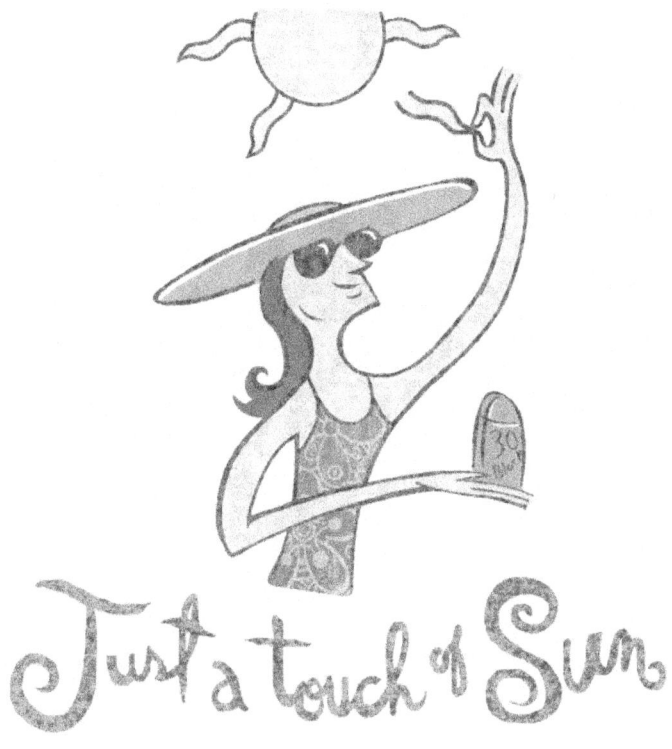

Just a touch of Sun

Rule #3

Allow Yourself Only a Touch of Sun

Sun gives us vitamin D, which is present in supplements and additives in milk but can be difficult to metabolize in these forms. The body *needs* sun and the Vitamin D it produces to aid in organ maintenance, calcium regulation and absorption, the immune system function, and bone formation. The mind also needs sun; it helps uplift the psyche.

However, despite some of the pleasurable and necessary benefits, too much sun causes skin cancer, hard and deep lines on the face, and macular degeneration in the eyes. It is okay to tan in the sun, but burning your skin causes elastin – the connective tissue in your skin, to deteriorate – to become less resilient. Elastin is what gives your skin the resilience and bounce that keeps wrinkles at bay (just as the name implies, it's like an elastic). But it frays when it is exposed to sun. So use **sunblock**. And while you're at it, protect your eyes with **sunglasses**. Wear a **hat** to further protect your eyes, face, and hair and to cut down on glare, which makes you squint.

Squinting is not only unattractive, it also causes more wrinkles.

When I was 13 years old, I bleached my hair without first reading the directions on the box. I left the bleach in overnight. My hair turned white. Then, over a three-week period, it all fell out. I was completely bald at age 13. Not a pretty sight for a gangly, insecure teenager.

Luckily, I went to ranch camp that summer in Wyoming where a cowboy hat all day was *de riguer*. At night I wore a stocking cap. By the summer's end I was packed off to boarding school with a fashionable pixie cut tipped in gold – very Mia Farrow looking. Mia, the doll of society and gossip columns, was dating Frank Sinatra at the time.

That experience taught me, by accident, the value of a **hat**. I love the shade for my eyes. It protects my skin from sun and glare. It protects my hair from wind and sun, which cause hair to dry out and become brittle.

My hair is still long – I never wore it short again once it grew out. It is still thick and lustrous because I take care of it. I wash it almost every day and I keep it brushed and tidy. I have it trimmed regularly and I wear it up or down, in pigtails or braids. I use hairspray. I have no favorite shampoo or conditioner – I use whatever is available.

The secret is the **HAT**.

Rule #4

Get Plenty of Sleep

If you feel sleepy during meetings, or while practicing yoga in the afternoon, chances are you are sleep deprived. Most of us are. We have jobs and families, we try to squeeze in exercise, we return phone calls and emails while preparing dinner, we wake ourselves early and go to bed late. There is almost no time to relax, and seemingly so little time to sleep.

But your mind and body need sleep to refresh the synapses and enable you to work at maximum capacity.

Everyone needs a different amount of sleep. If I go to bed at 11PM, I wake up without an alarm at 6AM. I need seven hours of sleep. On average, depending on their age, most people need somewhere between seven to eight hours of sleep each night. If you can't get the amount you need at night, find a way to take a nap during the day.

When I was a judge in New York City my brain would simply shut down at 3PM. I would put my head on my crossed arms on my desk and fall sound asleep for five to ten minutes. My boss, seeing this, would sometimes turn off my light and quietly close the door. She knew

I would wake up refreshed and able to work harder and even more efficiently.

Some people have trouble sleeping. One way to train your mind to get ready to sleep is to have a routine that triggers sleepiness. I read from 10:30 to 11PM. Boom. I'm sleepy. I turn off the light and I'm asleep in ten seconds. Watching TV to wind down and prepare for sleep **does not work**. TV seems to relax you, but actually it is stimulating enough to churn your brain into activity and keep you awake.

Meditation can be very helpful. The age-old counting sheep trick is really a form of meditation. Don't hang onto thoughts and don't try to problem solve. Just acknowledge any thoughts that come up, then release them. Allow the thoughts to float by like those sheep gracefully leaping over a fence. Relax and let your mind go into neutral.

You will sleep.

A good night's sleep refreshes you. It is so easy to feel overwhelmed when there aren't "enough hours in the day," and the tendency is to do just one more thing. But fatigue weakens your coping mechanisms. I have always found that going to bed when I'm tired rather than attempting to get everything done before I go to sleep enables me to be more refreshed and productive the next morning.

Sleep deprivation causes dark under-eye circles and puffiness, so you won't feel good with too little sleep, and you won't look good.

Make sleep a priority!

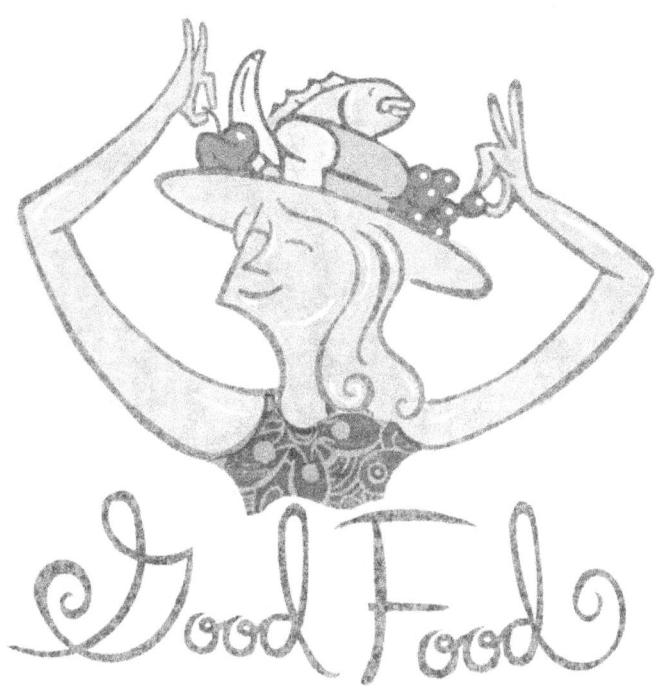

Good Food

Rule #5

Eat Good Food

Oh my, there are so many studies and stories about food. There is mad cow disease so we are afraid of serving beef for dinner, there is bird flu so we think twice or three times before eating chicken. There's mercury in fish, there are pesticides in veggies and fruits, and there's salmonella in eggs.

What *can* we eat?

The answer is: EVERYTHING.

However, eat in moderation. Stay away from fast food and packaged dinners; they are loaded with fats, sodium, and sugars. We get so busy with everyday life that we don't think we have time to cook a nice meal. We want to buy fast food as a quick fix.

This is okay maybe once a year but not once a week, much less once a day. Everybody likes their French fries now and then but eating such foods on a regular basis will very quickly take its toll.

You **do** have time to cook a meal. I wrote a cookbook called *Camp Cooking in the Adirondacks*, which outlines six basic meals that are easy to prepare after being out all day hiking or skiing or golfing or rowing my boat. It translates well for working families who all arrive home hungry after work and school.

Put the chicken in the oven, put the rice on, use frozen peas. While everything is cooking set the table, return a few phone calls, open your mail, and help your kids with their homework. When the meal is ready unplug the phone, light the candles, and all sit down together. Share the day with one another. You will be surprised at how rewarding this simple procedure is.

Remember: good food should be savored and enjoyed.

Eat lots of fruits and vegetables (locally grown if possible), eat whole grains such as rice, oatmeal, whole wheat bread, and quinoa. Eat free-range chicken, fresh fish from a good market, beef, lamb, pork, elk, and duck. Eat potatoes – they're loaded with vitamin K, which is good for your blood. I like to put butter on my potatoes but another great way to prepare them is sliced thick, drizzled with olive oil, and sprinkled with garlic powder and herbs. Bake them at 350 degrees for 30 minutes.

Broccoli and mushrooms are loaded with antioxidants – so are blueberries and pink grapefruit. Antioxidants fight cancer. It is always good to fend off a lurking enemy.

Garlic and hot pepper kill viruses and bacteria in your throat and gut. If you have a sore throat, take a tablespoon of hot sauce, such as Tabasco. Oh, you'll find it makes your eyes water, but the sting will go away and you won't get the cold.

Also good to keep in mind is that there are two different kinds of cholesterol: High Density Lipoproteins (HDL) are good because they cleans the blood vessels. You get HDL from cold-water fish such as shrimp, lobster, and clams.

Low Density Lipoprotein (LDL) is the bad kind of cholesterol because it clogs the blood vessels. LDL is present in butter, cream, fat on steak, or anything cooked in fat such as chicken nuggets or French fries. I have a particular penchant for heavy cream on my oatmeal and blueberries, so I stay away from fatty steaks and fast food. It's a worthwhile trade-off and it works because I keep my intake moderate.

"An apple a day keeps the doctor away." It's an old wives tale but it's true! The process of biting into the apple cleans the teeth and massages the gums. The tannic acid in the apple kills anaerobic bacteria that hide up in the gums and cause tooth decay and gum disease and, if virulent enough, can cause problems elsewhere. Apples contribute to overall health, which begins in the mouth.

Sweets are a special problem. Our primordial instincts, remaining from our days as cavemen, make our bodies think, "Sweet means ripe," so therefore it's good for you. But sugar, especially manufactured sugar, is not good. Cut down on it. It adds unnecessary calories, causing weight gain. It causes blood vessels to corrode. It contributes to the causes of diabetes, which is a dreadful disease.

Still, we crave sweets, so don't always deprive yourself. Just limit the amount. Have a small cookie for dessert instead of a large piece of cake. I carry a bag on M&M's with me most of the time. Three M&M's will satisfy me after lunch or dinner. Sometimes I order a cup of hot chocolate.

Now that's satisfying!

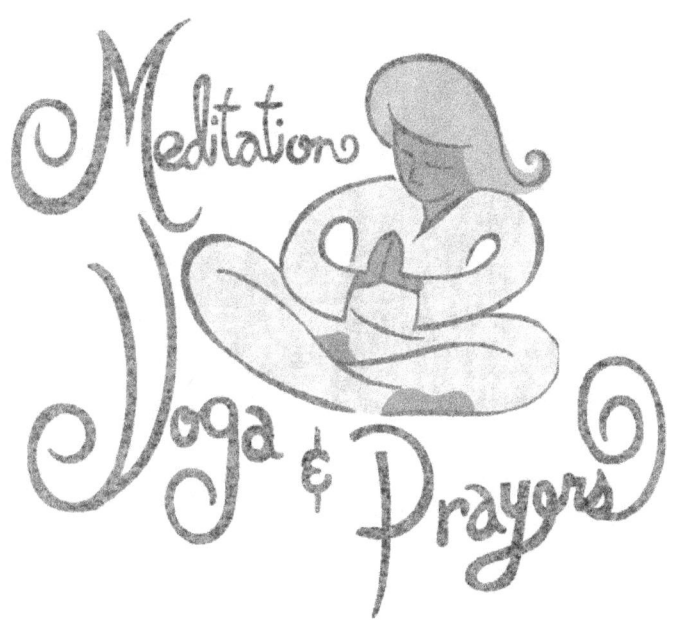

Rule #6

Meditate, Practice Yoga, Pray

These three elements comprise Rule #6 because they are each a form of focus. Individually and together they help eliminate extraneous distractions, and thus bring the body, the mind, and the spirit together to provide an empowering ability to concentrate and focus your thoughts and feelings, your goals and aspirations.

Meditation

There are techniques to help relax the brain entirely. I wrote earlier about meditation as a way to fall asleep. If you need sleep and you are meditating, you will probably fall asleep. But if you are well-rested, meditation will relax your mind while allowing inspirational thoughts to bubble forth. You will be empowered to do new and wonderful things. Meditation helps the body and mind attain harmony with one another.

Yoga

I take a yoga class every afternoon at 4PM. Our yoga master is a former drill instructor who found yoga was a way to heal broken body parts. Then he realized it was mentally healing as well. He quit West Point and went to an ashram and came out a yoga master. There are more men in my yoga class than women because they know the benefits of yoga stretching after exercise.

Yoga is not a competition with your neighbor, who may look like a pretzel or a graceful swan. Yoga is a conversation between you and your body. Do what is comfortable and never push hard enough to hurt yourself.

Many people in my class have had injuries or hip or knee replacements. They can't do some of the postures perfectly but they still take yoga for the overall benefits. Exercise bunches up the muscles, yoga stretches them out. Yoga helps with balance. Yoga centers your body. If you have an old injury – a bad knee or hip – you will favor it when you walk and stand, which means eventually you'll become lopsided in some way. The body will compensate for the pain and weakness by putting stress somewhere else.

I have a bad right knee from an old ski injury. Before I took yoga I had a nagging pain in my left hip. X-rays and scans showed no damage. It turned out that I was favoring my right leg and therefore stressing the left side of my body. With yoga, my body has re-aligned itself into a proper posture and the pain has subsided. With yoga and exercise the right knee is now almost as good as the left.

Prayer

We all need a way to not only relax the body and mind but to refresh the spirit. Prayer can be to the Great Spirit, or to Jesus, or to your favorite saint, or to God. It's another way to focus your thoughts.

When you are tempted to pray for that big job you're applying for, instead ask for strength, inspiration, and ability. Really, really focus on your own inner self to pull together what you need to move forward. You may not get that big job, but you will get the next one.

God does not push buttons. Praying is a way to integrate your mind and your emotions so you will perform at your best.

Focus.

And then let go.

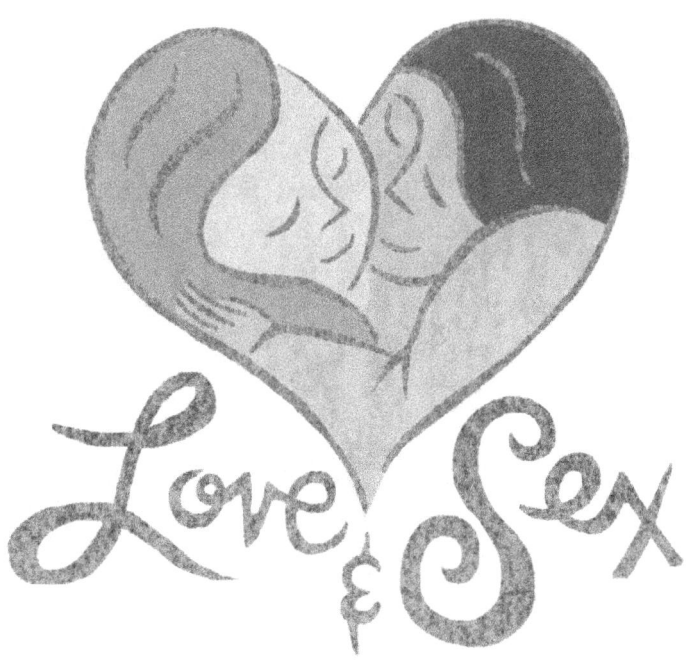

Rule #7

Love & Sex

It is a truly wonderful feeling to love someone totally and have good sex. Sex is a physical and emotional communion between two loving people.

It's possible to love someone and not have the sex. Love your spouse through illness or debilitating injuries. Maybe you're not married, or you have no "significant other," but you can still love. Love yourself! Love your friends, your children, your neighbor, your community, your pet.

When you love you are giving your best self to another person and in return you will receive 1,000 times what you give. But you must love totally, with abandon and without expectation of profit or gain.

What about sex without love? Not fulfilling. Don't go there. Get a vibrator.

You must have LOVE.

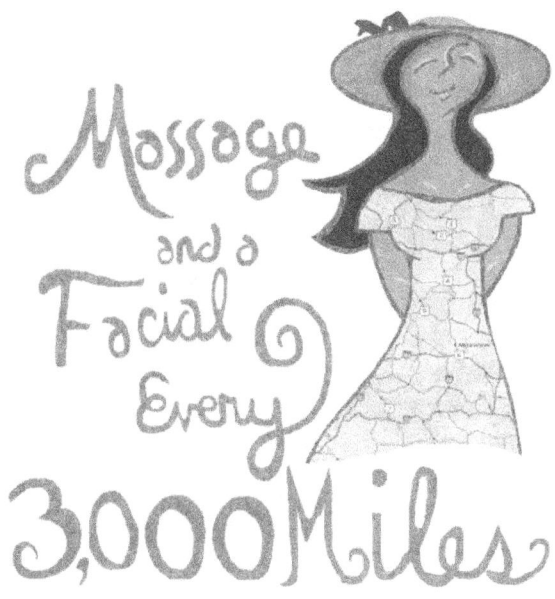

Rule #8

Have a Massage and a Facial Every 3,000 Miles

When I was a young bride in New York City we had an old Mercedes Benz. I would take it in for an oil change every 3,000 miles and it would cost almost $200. Eeek! That was a lot of money! I said to myself, "I'm worth at least as much as this car! I'm going to get a facial every time the car gets an oil change." So I have had regular facials every six to eight weeks for the last 40 years.

Facials

Facials not only relax those worry lines on your brow, they enrich and replenish your skin, clean the pores, and remove wayward hair. You benefit from taking a little nap while the mask works. After a rejuvenating hour you will walk out with clear, glowing skin and everyone will say, "Oh, you look so beautiful!" And, most facials cost less than that oil change.

Massage

While I was in law school I had a massage once a week. The massage relaxed me but also worked out the inevitable knots caused by stress and endless studying in odd poses. Now I have a massage about once a month. A good massage is a great way to release tension and **feel good**.

Go for it!

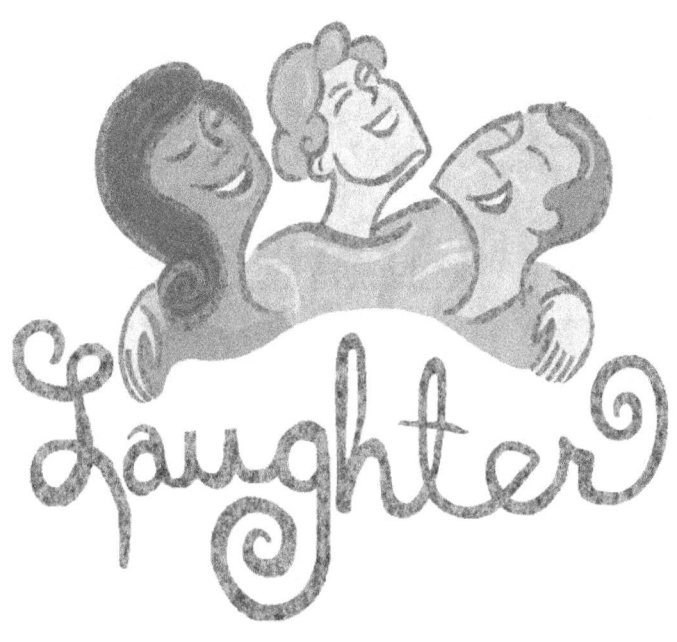

Rule #9
Laugh Often

Laughter not only feels good, it activates the immune system.

When I had a hysterectomy a friend gave me a Nancy Mitford novel about an English houseparty weekend. All the characters were so funny and got themselves into such crazy predicaments that the book had me laughing so hard that tears rolled down my cheeks.

I was discharged early. I had a quick recovery and no pain.

Laughter is a good way to uplift the spirit. Try to see the humor in every situation; laugh at it. Laugh at yourself. Laugh with your family and friends and your days will be joyous and fun. You will not only feel happier, you will be healthier. When you have to deal with an irritating situation put a big smile on your face and plow your way through it. You will find that physically smiling makes you smile from within, and makes you beautiful, too.

Smile!

Giggle!

Laugh!

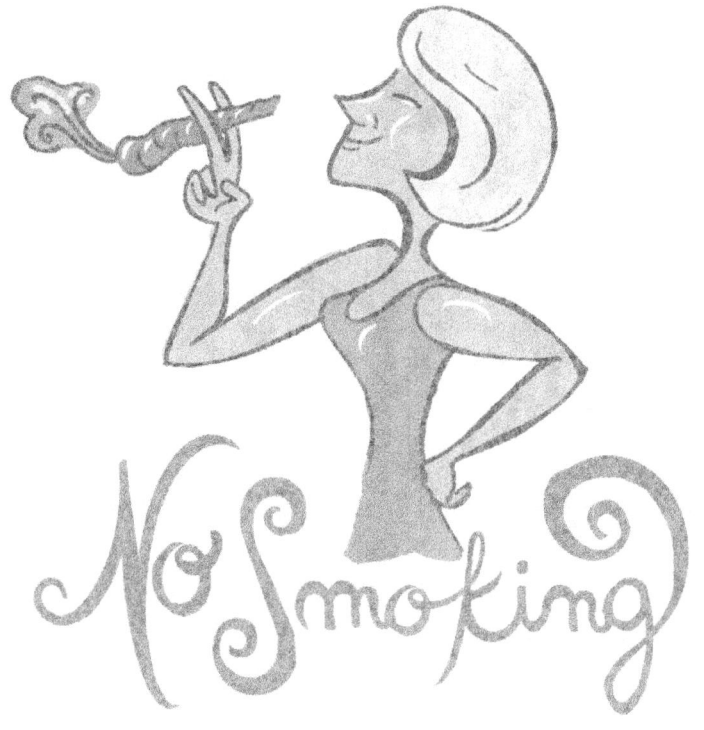

Rule #10

Do Not Smoke

Do I need to tell you how bad smoking is for you?

Smoking clogs the alveoli in the lungs so they are not able to efficiently transfer the incoming oxygen with the carbon dioxide trying to leave. The body **requires** oxygen. The body breathes out carbon dioxide as waste. Isn't it obvious that a pile of waste and not enough oxygen will negatively affect the overall functions of the body and mind, not to mention physical appearance?

Just think about how bad smoking can make your skin look. No matter how many facials you have, if you smoke your skin will show it – hard lines, grey pallor, loss of connective tissue. Smoking makes your breath smell awful and your clothes reek. Also, it can be an expensive habit.

Use the money you save by not smoking cigarettes to have regular massages and facials!

Nicotine and all the other chemicals they put in cigarettes are addictive, and you don't want to be addicted to anything but love.

Don't smoke!

Conclusion

Essentially the message of this book can be summed up in the following phrase:

Everything in moderation

Don't overdo any one thing, and remember this: everything in moderation, including moderation *but excluding love*. You can never have too much love!

Give love and get it.

Go forth and love.

A Note About the Author

Phebe Thorne is a registered nurse who graduated from Columbia University. A second career in politics led her to law school at Pace University in New York City, where she raised two sons and had a daughter at the end of her second school year. She went on to act as one of Mayor Rudolph Giuliani's "Quality of Life" judges until embarking on an athletic sabbatical to Sun Valley, where she now spends the majority of her year skiing, snow-shoeing, practicing yoga, and participating in the Court Appointed Special Advocates (CASA) program. Each summer she resides in the Adirondacks, where her family camp is tucked away in the splendor of the world's oldest mountains. There she golfs, entertains with delightful grace and ease, and rows her 19th-century guideboat.

Between her migrations and her active schedules, Phebe has written a cookbook titled *Camp Cooking in the Adirondacks*. Her second book, *Massage and a Facial Every 3,000 Miles*, is soon to be followed by a third: *A History of the Uplands: Life in a Living Museum*.

Stay tuned.